FIVE HERBAL TEA RECIPES THAT WILL BALANCE YOUR LIFE

I0163924

Nutrient, health benefits,

and

fun facts on all ingredients

Stephen T. Radentz

Disclaimer

I am not a doctor. I am not giving health advice. I am just giving you some basic facts about some extremely healthy plants. The information contained in this report is for general information and educational purposes only. It does not constitute medical advice. Therefore, any reliance you place on such information is strictly at your own risk. Please check with your medical doctor before starting or changing your medical routine.

Thank you, Christine, my wife for showing me the way. You brought herbs, and then tea into my life. That simple act has changed my life dramatically.
Thank you, I love you.

TEA BLENDS

BALANCED BLEND	ENERGY & FOCUS
Lemon Balm	Ashwagandha
Holy Basil	Orange Peel
St. John's Wort	Lemon Balm
Rosehip	Yerba Mate
Rose Petal	Green Tea
Orange Peel	
IMMUNE BOOSTER	**COLD & FLU**
Elderberry	Echinacea
Ginger	Holy Basil
Elderflower	Ginger
Holy Basil	Lemongrass
Lemon Peel	Green Tea
Blue or Blackberry	Elderberry
SLEEP & RELAXATION	
Valerian Root	Spearmint
Lavender	Chamomile
Passionflower	

Introduction

Herbal tea is one of the most nutritious drinks available today. It is easy to blend yourself, or there is a plethora of readymade varieties as well. Health experts the world over recommend that you drink 64 ounces of water every day. That is some exceptionally good advice. Staying hydrated will keep your body balanced and ready for the next adventure. However, what if instead of just plain water, you drank an herbal iced tea? Not only will you be hydrated, but you would also be blasting your body with a variety of must have nutrients.

Once I started drinking around 60 ounces of herbal cold tea a day, my body, mind, and energy level improved. I have a more focused and balanced feeling throughout my day. I accomplished more because my energy level remains high. I feel good all day because I am replenishing vital nutrients throughout the day. I guarantee that my body has what it needs for whatever I encounter.

On the following pages you will find five amazing herbal blends that will balance, calm, energize, improve immunities and your health, and help you sleep better. You will not only get some amazing recipes I will also provide the health benefits that each of the ingredients provide you, and a general description of the effects of how each blend can be expected to make you feel.

You'll even get some history, and some other interesting trivia about some amazing herbs.

There are studies that are beginning to prove that when you know how a vitamin is supposed to react with your body, the health benefits get multiplied. It appears that knowing what to expect, increases the benefit of the nutrients. I recommend that you read the whole recipe and learn how the different herbs will work with your body as you make the tea blend. This way you are programming your mind how you want the herbs to help you. Sounds kinda far out, I know. But trust me and give it a try.

All the herbs listed have many micronutrients, phytonutrients, flavonoids, and other nutrients not mentioned in the report including omega 3 and 6. Most of the herbs have high amounts of antioxidant abilities as well. I have tried to pick herbs that target the three life centers: the head, chest, and the gut. This creates a balancing effect in your body, as well as receiving individual benefits from each herb.

I highly recommend adding herbal teas to your diet.

Drink in the benefits.

Balanced Blend

Below you will find one of my favorite blends of herbal tea. All the ingredients affect your life centers, the head, chest, and gut. This blend can not only make you healthier, but it can also increase blood circulation, reduce stress, anxiety, and depression, while removing toxins from your blood. It will help your body become balanced.

I use this blend about 3 times a week.

Ingredients

- *lemon balm*
- *Holy basil*
- *St. John's wort*
- *Rosehip*
- *Rose petals*
- *Orange peel*

Instructions:

- Blend 1 tsp of each herb into a tea strainer. You can use cheesecloth, or tea bags as well. If filling your own tea bags mix herbs together first, then fill bags with the blend.

- Soak in ½ gallon of water (distilled water is best) for 6 to 12 hours.
- Remove herb packet and serve.
- Makes ½ gallon of tea.

You can use the same herbs for a second soak that will be a little less flavorful. I will sometimes add 2 green or black tea bags during the second soaking to boost flavor and health benefits. *Makes ½ gallon of tea.*Individual tea bags will make 6-8 oz.

Lemon Balm: Melissa officinalis

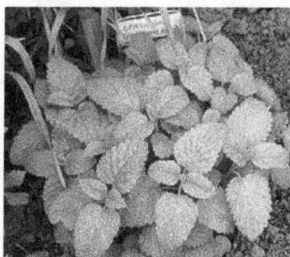

BENEFITS:

Relieves stress and anxiety, improves brain functions and memory, improves lung functions, reduces blood pressure, improves digestion, supports liver and kidney functions.

NUTRIENTS:

Vitamins A & C, Iron, Calcium, Potassium, Magnesium, Zinc.

One of my favorite "balancing herbs". Lemon balm has an amazing smell and will also affect your three life centers. It is great for maintaining full body balance (Homeostasis). Lemon balm can be used daily with no known negative side effects. Used alone it will make a great hot, or iced tea. You can cook with it to add color and taste to any dish, it is easily extracted in olive and coconut oil. Feel free to soak it in oil for thirty days, and you now have lemon balm infused oil.

The leaves have a subtle lemony flavor that reminds me of lemon candy from the 1980's. When the plant is processed it releases this amazing lemon scent that just fills the room with a fresh clean scent.

Lemon balm has been used for over three thousand years. The Greeks and Romans used it as a medicine and as a spice. The Roman emperor Charlemagne was so grateful for Lemon Balm's calming effect, he stated every healing garden should include this amazing herb due to its medicinal benefits. Lemon balm, in case you didn't know, is a member of the mint family. Looking at the leaves you can see the similarity. Unsurprisingly, lemon balm can be used to freshen your breath.

Tulsi (Holy Basil): Ocimum sanctum L

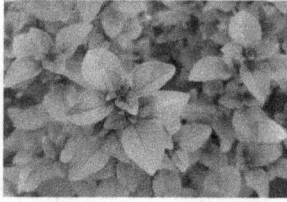

BENEFITS:

Improves brain functions, reduces stress, enhances metabolism, improves digestion, and reduces stomach acid. Lowers blood sugar, improves circulation. It is high in antioxidants and is an anti-inflammatory.

NUTRIENTS:

Vitamins A, C, & K. Iron, Calcium, Zinc. Manganese.
Dried basil has 43% RDA of vitamin K, whereas fresh has approximately 5%.

Holy basil is a super balancing herb that affects your whole body in a positive way. This variety of basil has more nutrients than all other basil varieties (Ocimum Sanctum L). It is considered the most medicinal of the genus. (similarly, cannabis is more medicinal than hemp, yet they are of the same family of plant)

A primary action of holy basil is its ability to bring down fevers. During a deadly outbreak of viral encephalitis in Northern India in 1978, holy basil was compared with standard

10

conventional treatments. At a dose of only 2.5 grams of holy basil powder taken four times daily, there was complete recovery in 60 percent of the patients using the herb, contrasted with a survival rate of zero of those treated with conventional medicine. Tulsi is also a member of the mint family (Lamiaceae) and is native to India and southeast Asia where it has been used in Ayurvedic medicine for centuries. Holy basil is an extremely important herb in the Hindu religion. Its origin can be traced back to the very beginning of the religion and is associated with their God's. Tulsi can be found growing throughout India both in personal gardens and in temples for its spiritual and health benefits. A super herb that will maintain balance in your body.

St. John's wort: Hypericum perforatum

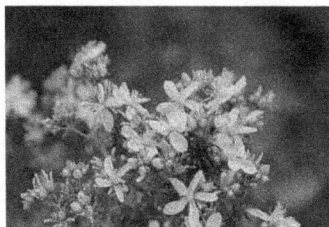

BENEFITS:

Anti-depressant, (proven to be as effective as Prozac/Fluoxetine). May release serotonin which makes you happy. reduces anxiety, improves blood circulation, antiviral, and may improve digestion.

NUTRIENTS:
Vitamins A & C, carotenoids, tannins, hypericin and pseudo hypericin.

Wow! What can I say, an amazing all-natural antidepressant? (has been proven to be as effective as Prozac) This is one of my extreme "balancing Herbs" because it affects all three life centers. It helps to keep your body balanced. Most herbs have this effect, but St. John's Wort is a body balancing bomb. It has been used medicinally for over two thousand years. The Greeks were one of the first nations to document using it in the 1st century. (the Greeks took many ideas from Egypt, so my guess is that SJW use as medicine is much older).

SJW improves your liver's ability to process chemicals. (funny how a bad thing about SJW is that it helps your body work at a higher level.) Improved liver function is only a bad thing if you mix it with "man-made" synthetic medicine.

If you are taking prescription drugs (you shouldn't), but if you must take synthetic medicine, check with your doctor, as St. John's Wort may have an effect on the medication, because your liver will function at a higher level. Your improved liver mixed with prescription drugs may not be good for you so ask your doctor if medicating with an herb would be ok.

Rosehip: Rosa canina, R. gallica, R. rugosa, R. villosa

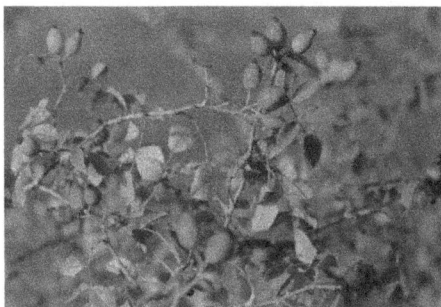

BENEFITS:

Improves immune system, high in antioxidants, anti-inflammatory, stimulates white blood cell production, and reduces blood pressure. Improves gut health. Supports the heart, as well as strengthens the immune system.

NUTRIENTS:

Vitamins A, C, E and B6, Potassium, Calcium, Iron, Magnesium.

Rosehip is one of my go to herbs for vitamin C. It has more than an orange. If fresh fruit is unavailable, adding rosehip will provide the vitamin C boost your body needs.

Rosehip or Rose haws have been used since ancient times for their healing properties. The first known cultivators were the Persians and use of the berries spread from Persia to Rome and Greece. Today many cultures still use the fruit as a folk medicine. In 77 AD, Roman writer Pliny the Elder recorded more than 30 different medicinal uses for the rose plant and its berries, and in the middle age's rosehips were used to make Catholic rosaries and incorporated into worship ceremonies, giving the fruit religious significance. Rosehips were gathered for their vitamin C content to support the war effort during WWII, as fresh fruit was in short supply.

As you can see, the rosehip can bring some amazing health benefits to your body. They may not be as pretty to look at as the flowers, but the nutrients available will boost your body to good health.

Rose petals: *Rosa; L*

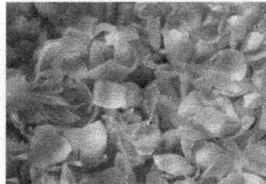

BENEFITS:

Increases good bacteria in the gut, improves digestion, removes toxins in blood, boosts the immune system, is high in antioxidants, antidepressant, improves brain functions. Has antibacterial, antiviral, and anti-inflammatory properties.

NUTRIENTS:
Vitamins A, C, E and B6, Potassium, Calcium, Iron, Magnesium

As with rosehip, rose petals have similar health benefits. With a plethora of antioxidants and anthocyanins, rose petals can assist your body in fighting off cancers.

Rose petals have also been used since man began using plants as medicine. Their use continues today in tea, tinctures, lotions, and in everyday meals. Roses have been found in fossilized materials dating back 35 million years ago. Drawings of rose petals being used as medicine, and as decoration have also been found in Egyptian pyramids. It is believed that early cultivation began 5000 years ago in China and Egypt, and then spread to the world via the silk road.

I like the scent they give of as well as their soothing taste. It creates just a subtle flavor that is refreshing. Breathing in the aroma also provides you with a calming anti-anxiety effect.

Orange peel: *Citrus Sinensis*

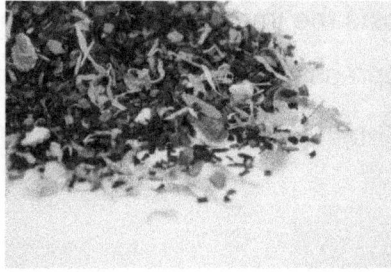

BENEFITS:

High vitamin C, high in antioxidants, improves brain functions, improves digestion, anti-inflammatory, lowers blood pressure, boosts immune system.

NUTRIENTS:

Vitamins A, B6, C, and E. Calcium, Iron, Magnesium, Phosphorus, Potassium, zinc, and copper.

Orange peel use can be traced back 7000 years to India where it was used in cooking. The fruit then spread to Asia and then to Europe where it was then brought to the Americas.

Today oranges can be found on almost every continent. The world produces on average 50 million tons of oranges a year. America harvests around 4 million tons a year, mostly from California. May 4th is national candied orange peel day (believe it or not) and is celebrated by making, and eating sugar and honey covered orange peels. The practice goes back to ancient time in the middle east and Asia, where the sugary treats were used to decorate cakes and other sweet dishes.

An orange's high vitamin C content is the most obvious health benefit. However, the orange is full of nutrients that when consumed, they all work together for your body's benefit. It is not just vitamin C that heals you, it is all the nutrients working together with you that creates the healing effect of oranges and all other natural foods.

Orange peel will add a citrus flavor to your tea. Creating that tropical feeling you get when you think of oranges. Great additional health blast for your body.

Cold and flu blend

This awesome herbal blend will not only assist your body to perform better, but it will also reduce your body's exposure to viral and bacterial germs. How can this be, you ask? The herbs chosen all have anti-viral as well as antibacterial properties, and they are high in antioxidants, (cancer / zombie cell busters).

What this means for you is that you are putting good antibodies in your body that will be able to fight back against disease. Maintaining the correct nutrients in your body is imperative when fighting off sickness. The right nutrients, plus positive momentum will keep you healthy.

This awesome herbal tea blend will be your partner in fighting back against colds and flu.

Ingredients

- *Echinacea*
- *Holy basil*
- *Ginger*
- *Lemongrass*
- *Green tea*
- *Elderberry*

Instructions:

- Blend 1 tsp of each herb into a tea strainer. You can use cheesecloth, or tea bags as well. If filling your own tea bags mix herbs together first, then fill bags with the blend.
- Soak in ½ gallon of water (distilled water is best) for 6 to 12 hours.
- Remove herb packet and serve.
- Makes ½ gallon of tea.

You can use the same herbs for a second soak that will be a little less flavorful. I will sometimes add 2 green or black tea bags during the second soaking to boost flavor and health benefits. *Makes ½ gallon of tea.*Individual tea bags will make 6-8 oz.

Echinacea: *Echinacea angustifolia and Echinacea purpurea*

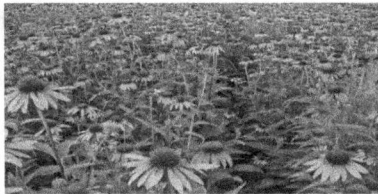

BENEFITS:

Anti-inflammatory, antioxidant, and antiviral properties, immune strengthening. Fights colds and flu. Controls blood sugar, high in antioxidants that promote healthy cell growth.

NUTRIENTS:

Vitamins A & C, Calcium, Zinc, Iron

Echinacea, also referred to as coneflower or purple coneflower is native to North America and Canada. The origin of the medicinal use of the plant is unknown. However, it is known that native Americans used echinacea for hundreds maybe thousands of years. The indigenous people of America used the rootstalk for medicine to treat many ailments. Colds, virus, pain, and inflammation. It was even used to treat saddle sores on horses.

Today there are over 400 scientific studies mostly agreeing with the health claims. Echinacea is an awesome cold buster and I begin taking it weekly or more in September, the beginning of cold and flu season. I just figure you might as well have the best cold fighting nutrients in your body before the virus attacks. However, echinacea use should not be for every day. Your body will become saturated with the nutrients, and they can lose their effectiveness. I believe that using it once or twice a week during flu season provides excellent protection from viruses. If you feel. A cold or flu coming on you can use echinacea up to a week every day, then take a break for a few days and let your body have time to absorb the nutrients before using it again.

Echinacea has been proven by millions of personal case studies to assist you in preventing or reducing a viral attack. One of my favorite herbs for anti-cold.

Holy Basil (Tulsi): *Ocimum sanctum L*

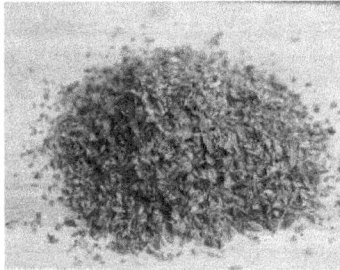

BENEFITS:

Antimicrobial, antibacterial, antiviral, antifungal, antidiarrheal, Antioxidant, anti-inflammatory, liver, brain and heart protectant, antidiabetic, antipyretic antitussive, (treats cough), anti-arthritic, Anti-coagulant, apoptogenic, stress reducer.

NUTRIENTS:

Vitamins A, C, & K. Iron, Calcium, Zinc. Manganese. *Dried Tulsi has 43% RDA of vitamin K, whereas fresh basil has approximately 5%.*

As stated, earlier Tulsi is an amazing healing, life giving plant. It can be consumed every day with little to no negative side effects (similar to cannabis).

This herb is the power punch for your three life centers, the head, chest, and the gut. Tulsi assists in maintaining balanced blood sugar levels, as well as stress hormones. It positively affects the central nervous system and blood circulation. Holy basil also calms your stomach acid which aids in digestion. Tulsi will also assist in keeping the respiratory system functioning at a high level.

It is the one herb I recommend for daily use. There are studies that show Tulsi even has anticancer benefits. It is so beneficial for you! One of my favorite herbs, it balances the body while promoting optimal health. an amazing life-giving herb.

Ginger: *Zingiber officinale*

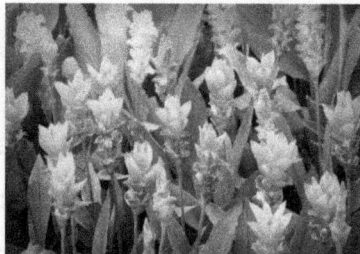

BENEFITS:

Antiviral, anti-bacterial, anti-inflammatory, anti-nausea. Ginger improves circulation, lowers blood sugar, and is loaded with antioxidants.

NUTRIENTS:
Vitamin B6, & C, Potassium, Magnesium. Manganese,

Ginger has been used in Chinese medicine for thousands of years as an immunity booster. It has been found in artifacts in southeast Asia dating over 5000 years old. It was found in medicine bags carried by local tribes. It is not known to grow in the wild, and it appears to have always been cultivated.

Ginger, Galangal, and Turmeric, are all similar root plants. We use the rhizomes either dried or fresh in cooking, tea, lotions, etc. Any of the mentioned root plants may be substituted for this recipe. For a mild ginger flavor, I recommend trying Galangal (Thai ginger). It has all the benefits with less spicy flavor.

On a side note, these plants are easy to grow in containers. if you are limited on your available growing space an 8"- 12' container would bring you a nice sized harvest. Simply take the ginger root, place the little knobs facing up, and keep moist. Maybe add a little balanced fertilizer at the beginning, and then again at three months. Ginger is a fairly easy plant to grow.

Lemongrass: *Cymbopogon*

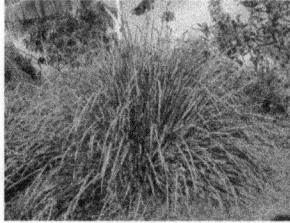

BENEFITS: Antibacterial, antiviral anti-inflammatory, antimicrobial, immune and blood booster. May improve digestion and reduce risk of cancer.

NUTRIENTS:
Vitamins A & C, Calcium, Potassium, Magnesium, Manganese, iron

Lemongrass, also referred to as *fever grass* due to its fever reducing ability has been used for centuries like most other herbs. The plant has long stalks that are like saw grass only not as sharp. The plant's origins stem from Asia where it has been, and still is used in foods and medicine regularly.

Like holy basil, lemongrass is grown all over India. As a matter of fact, India produces 80% of the world's commercial lemongrass. It can be eaten, used in lotions, and it has also become a favorite aromatherapy fragrance that creates a calm relaxed feeling at a fraction of the price of other calming essential oils. It may even help reduce headaches.

The fragrance, like lemon balm, has an amazing fresh lemony scent, and when processing the leaves indoors, it will fill your house with the scent of lemon.

Green Tea: *Camellia Sinensis*

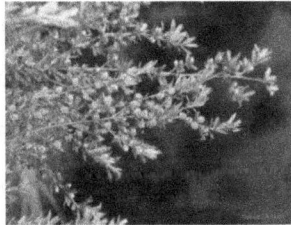

BENEFITS:

Improves brain function, antibacterial, antiviral, anti-inflammatory, regulates metabolism, antioxidant,

NUTRIENTS:

vitamins A, B, C and D. Potassium, Phosphorus, Manganese, Zinc

The search for the origin of green tea is a challenge. There are several legends claiming the truth all beginning around 3000 BC. Here's a crazy coincidence. Similar to the origin of black tea, green tea was discovered by an accident involving an army in China. The closest to the truth we think, is that Chinese emperor Shennong was traveling and stopped to camp for the night with his armies. A few camellia sinensis leaves, or flowers fell into the cup of water he was drinking. He liked the flavor so much that he sent soldiers to find the tree and collect the leaves. And that's how we believe green tea was born.

Several studies have shown that green tea has cancer fighting capabilities. It has been called the healthiest drink on the planet by many sources. It can improve memory, brain functions, and mood. Green tea has been shown to have more antioxidants than many so-called superfoods. It even has anti-aging benefits and it's great for your skin.

Although green tea has less caffeine than black tea, or coffee, it does provide a sense of alertness by increasing your metabolism. Enjoying all the health benefits in green tea will help you feel more positive, which will aid in healing your body faster.

Elderberry: *Sambucus nigra / canadensis*

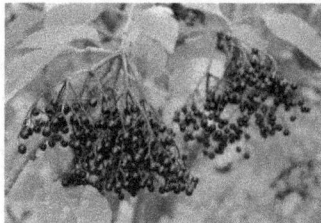

BENEFITS:

High in anthocyanins and antioxidants, antiviral antibacterial, anti-inflammatory. Relieves cold and flu symptoms and may also shorten the duration of colds. Improves kidney function and relieves stress. Great cold and flu season herb!

NUTRIENTS:

Vitamins A, B6, C, Phosphorus, Magnesium, Calcium, Potassium, Iron.

WOW, elderberries are certainly a super herb. They are in the spotlight as a cold and flu fighting powerhouse of natural medicine. Here's an excerpt from wikipedia.org: "Elderberry contains a unique compound called Antivirin® that can help protect healthy cells and inactivate infectious viruses. When given to patients, scientists have found the Black Elderberry has the ability to ward off flu infections quickly (Zakay-Rones 2004)". We can trace the medicinal use of elderberry back to ancient Egypt, however the famous Greek physician Hippocrates called elderberry his "medicine chest", because he used it for so many maladies. Elderberries are the gold standard of cold, flu and antiviral herbs. Elderberry syrup (a combination of thyme, elderberries, orange, and honey) is an amazing cold prevention medicine. Taking the syrup for three days is usually enough to stop the cold or flu in its tracks. Many people swear by eating vitamin C when they feel a cold coming on. However, consuming all of the nutrients in elderberries will not only help prevent an illness, but it will also many times stop an illness within 2 or 3 days.

Today as epidemics and pandemic viruses continue to spring up, elderberries are once again becoming a staple in our war chest for health.

Energized Focus Blend

Here is an herbal tea blend that will give you energy and heightened awareness, without anxiety or the jitters. This blend contains herbs that will increase your energy, and yes, some have natural caffeine, while other herbs assist your body to balance the jittery effect of the caffeine. This allows your body to be balanced, while your mind is free and energized to get the work done. Unlike synthetic energy drinks and pills, when drinking this blend of herbs will not only give you energy, focus and clarity. It will also be promoting good health in your body. Herbs are body balancing plants, you can get specific results, but at the same time the herbs are positively affecting your entire body... Balanced by Nature.

Ingredients

- *Ashwagandha*
- *Orange peel*
- *Lemon balm*
- *Yerba Mate*
- *Green tea*

Instructions:

- Blend 1 tsp of each herb into a tea strainer. You can use cheesecloth, or tea bags as well. If filling your own tea bags mix herbs together first, then fill bags with the blend.
- Soak in ½ gallon of water (distilled water is best) for 6 to 12 hours.
- Remove herb packet and serve.
- Makes ½ gallon of tea.

You can use the same herbs for a second soak that will be a little less flavorful. I will sometimes add 2 green or black tea bags during the second soaking to boost flavor and health benefits. *Makes ½ gallon of tea.*Individual tea bags will make 6-8 oz.

Ashwagandha: *Withania somnifera*

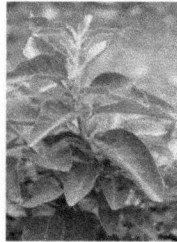

BENEFITS:
Reduces stress, improves brain functions, and calms the mind. Anti-inflammatory, antioxidant, antibacterial, anti-cancer,

antidepressant. Improves mood, increases focus, and is an immune booster.

NUTRIENTS:
Vitamins C & B, Calcium, Iron.

Ashwagandha, also referred to as *Winter cherry,* or *Indian ginseng,* is an apoptogenic herb that nourishes the adrenal glands and central nervous system. This one herb provides energy while it calms you. High in antioxidants it creates a healthy balanced environment for your body. Excellent choice for staying calm, energized, focused, and happy.

Ashwagandha has been used in India for over 6000 years in Ayurveda medicine. Ashwa means smells like horse, and ghanda means strength. And that is how it got its name. Ashwagandha on consuming it, it will give you the power of a smelly horse. Not entirely true, the plant does not smell like a horse. It is really another life-giving herb.

The entire plant can be used including the roots. Each part of the plant provides a variety of benefits to your body. Using the whole plant will assist your body in reaching homeostasis. The roots are normally ground into a powder, and then blended in water as a tea. Many people also add the powder to their smoothie, boosting the other ingredients. The leaves and stalk may also be used medicinally.

Ashwagandha may be used as a stand-alone ingredient for tea or added to a blend like this. Another super herb that balances your entire body.

Yerba Mate: *Ilex paraguariensis*,

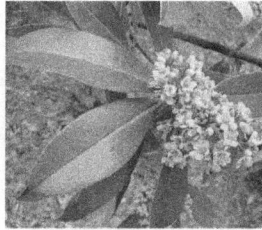

BENEFITS:

Xanthine's: *These compounds act as stimulants. They include caffeine and theobromine, which are also found in tea, coffee, and chocolate.* Anti-inflammatory, high in antioxidants, increases energy, focus, and mood. Lowers blood sugar and boosts the immune system.

NUTRIENTS:

vitamins B1, B2 and C, Phosphorus, Potassium, Magnesium, Manganese, Iron, Calcium

Approximately 80mg of caffeine per 8 oz. Similar to coffee.

The origins of yerba mate, Pronounced, *sher bah mah-tay*, comes from the Guaraní natives of pre-Columbian Paraguay and South America. These indigenous people had been using the plant as medicine for centuries. The plant leaves are dried and then used in tea. The locals drink the tea from special "mate" gourds created just for the purpose of enjoying the drink.

Around 1600 as Spanish conquerors arrived in South America the herb was used in trade and began to gain popularity as a coffee substitute. Today over 800,000 tons of Yerba Mate are harvested primarily in Argentina and Paraguay.

Yerba Mate can help with digestion, it promotes good bacteria growth in the gut. It lowers blood pressure and may improve circulation. Another amazing balancing herbs.

This is a great energy boosting herb that brings health benefits as well. However, it is recommended that you limit how often you drink it. Consumed in large quantities it may be connected to contributing to mouth cancer although I have found limited studies to validate this.

Orange peel: *Citrus Sinensis*

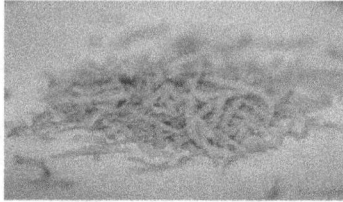

BENEFITS:

Lowers blood pressure, boosts the immune system, anti-inflammatory, regulates blood sugar. High in vitamin C and other nutrients. Contains a good number of antioxidants, flavonoids, and phytonutrients.

NUTRIENTS:

Vitamins A, B6, C, and E. Calcium, Iron, Magnesium, Phosphorus, Potassium, zinc, and copper.

Orange peel use can be traced back 7000 years to India where it was used in cooking. The fruit then spread to Asia and then to Europe where it was then brought to the Americas. It is believed that Columbus first brought seeds from Spain and had them planted in Haiti.

Today oranges can be found on almost every continent. The world produces on average 50 million tons of oranges a year. America harvests around 4 million tons a year, mostly from California.

Their high vitamin C content is the most obvious health benefit. However, the orange is full of nutrients that when consumed, they all work together for your body's benefit. It is not just vitamin C that heals you, it is all the nutrients working together with you that creates the healing effect of oranges. Orange peels may have a few more nutrients than oranges. The micronutrients are responsible for the anti-cancer and anti-inflammatory benefits. They are also responsible for helping clear our lungs allowing us to breathe more freely.

Orange peel will add a citrus flavor to your tea. Creating that tropical feeling you get when you think of oranges. Great additional health blast for your body.

Lemon Balm: *Melissa officinalis*

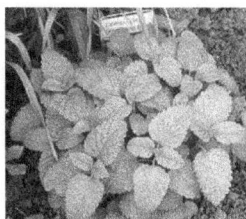

BENEFITS:

Anti-anxiety and stress reducer. Provides balance to your body by interacting with your head, chest, and gut, your life centers. It can also boost brain function, improves digestion, and can relieve nausea.

NUTRIENTS:
Vitamins A, C, Iron, Calcium, Potassium, Magnesium, Zinc.

Lemon balm, also known as Bee balm, Sweet balm, and sometimes even Honey plant, is an amazing herb that will bring an assortment of nutrients to your three life centers. Another amazing balancing herb that calms and balances the body and mind allowing you to relax. It has been used for centuries to bring a calm feeling, enabling the user to fall asleep. However, as it calms it does not bring a "drowsy" feeling. The sedative action of lemon balm is due to the presence of rosmarinic acid, which inhibits an enzyme involved in the triggering symptoms of anxiety and other mood disorders called GABA transaminase. However, this means that lemon balm may increase the effect of anti-anxiety medications, so the two should never be combined. Consult your doctor if you have any concerns. This calming yet alert effect allows us to use lemon balm to be calm but not sleepy.

It has been successfully studied that lemon balm can increase cognitive skills, and boost memory. It has also been used to reduce headaches, lower blood pressure, and can improve digestion. It works with your entire body.

When lemon balm is allowed to flower honeybees will flock to the nectar. It seems that the bees understand plant medicine, and realize just how nutritious, and beneficial the plant is.

Lemon balm is a plant for royalty as King Charles V of France regularly drank lemon balm tea for its health and anti-aging benefits. As noted, earlier King Charlemagne issued an edict that during his reign (of 47 years) every citizen of France should grow lemon balm in their gardens. He felt the healing benefits would be good for his population, and he was right.

So, you can see that lemon balm is an amazing balancing herb that has been used for thousands of years. Even bees know how beneficial lemon balm is. That is why I use it regularly in many different tea blends. Safe enough for everyday use, but remember, variety and moderation will allow you to reach perfect homeostasis.

Black tea: Camellia sinensis

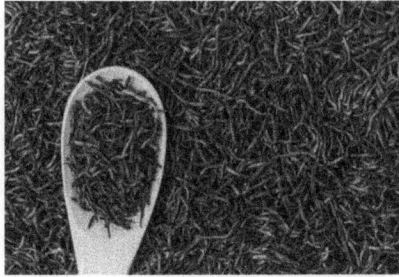

BENEFITS:

High in antioxidants, improves heart and gut health. Improves circulation and blood sugar levels, energy booster (caffeine), anticancer, and stress reducer.

NUTRIENTS:

Potassium, Magnesium, Phosphorus,
One cup contains 47mg caffeine.

Here is a crazy fact, black tea was most likely discovered in China due to an accident. Teas are graded on the processing method, and it is believed that during the Ming dynasty the tea was over oxidized (dried) and Wala, black tea was created. Apparently, an army had camped at the tea processing facility which caused a delay in processing the leaves. To save the harvest the farmer then smoked the leaves to complete the process and save the harvest. Today black tea is the most popular variety, and around 80% of the tea consumed is black.

Black tea has the highest amounts of caffeine of all tea. I included it to give you energy to get through the day. Black tea does not give me the caffeine jitters that coffee does, meaning I can drink it at any time of the day or night. However, I would not recommend drinking this blend near bedtime. You could always remove the black tea and replace it with chamomile for a relaxing nighttime blend.

Sleepy Time Tea

A perfect blend of powerhouse resting herbs. Chamomile tea is great by itself as a sleep aid. The below blend will bring sleep while calming and healing the body.

Ingredients

- *Valerian root*
- *Lavender*
- *Passionflower*
- *Spearmint*
- *Chamomile*

Instructions:

- Blend 1 tsp of each herb into a tea strainer. You can use cheesecloth, or tea bags as well. If filling your own tea bags mix herbs together first, then fill bags with the blend.
- Soak in ½ gallon of water (distilled water is best) for 6 to 12 hours.
- Remove herb packet and serve.
- Makes ½ gallon of tea.

You can use the same herbs for a second soak that will be a little less flavorful. I will sometimes add 2 green or black tea bags during the second soaking to boost flavor and health benefits. *Makes ½ gallon of tea.*Individual tea bags will make 6-8 oz.

Valerian root: *Valeriana officinalis*

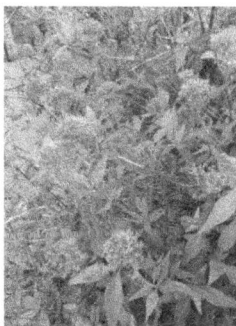

BENEFITS:

Proven to be a sleep aid. Calms anxiety improves nerve communication with the brain causing a balancing effect on your body. Antioxidant, anti-stress, Anti-anxiety .

NUTRIENTS:

Calcium, (valerenic acid and valenol, valepotriates, and a few alkaloids, actinidine, chatinine, shyanthine, valerianine, and valerine)

Native to Europe and parts of Asia, Valerian root has been called "nature's Valium", and it is one of the best choices for your health. It has been used since ancient times to promote calm and improve sleep. Interestingly, the name "valerian" is derived from the Latin verb valere, which means "to be strong" or "to be healthy."

Historically valerian root has been used to treat Insomnia, anxiety, and headaches, Hippocrates the father of modern medicine, documented using valerian to treat headaches, nervousness, trembling, and heart palpitations. Another amazing herb that has been successfully used for centuries to keep us healthy.

Valerian is a powerful calming herb. It is also an excellent natural antidepressant, could most likely be a great choice to calm hyperactivity in ADD and ADHD sufferers. Most known for its proven and documented success in treating insomnia it has become a *standalone* sleep aid. Combined with these other herbs prepare yourself for a relaxing, health restoring, sound sleep.

Lavender: *Lavandula*

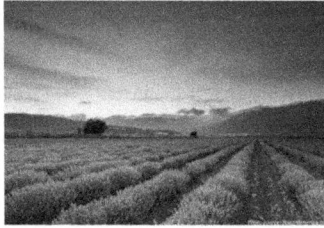

BENEFITS:

Stress reducer, calming, relieves headache pain. Improves digestion and relieves nausea. Calms nerve communication in the brain bringing a relaxing, sleepy feeling. Boosts your immune system which helps you heal while you sleep.

NUTRIENTS:

Vitamins A & C, Calcium, Iron.

Lavender is one of my favorite flowers, I have always wanted 20 or 30 acres of blooming lavender plants. Such a cool sight. The lavender plant not only is beautiful to look at, but it also has a plethora of health benefits for us as well. Its use dates to ancient Egypt where it was used in the preparation of mummies. It was also used in Rome in public bath houses, as well as for medicine, and as a fragrance. In the 17th century lavender processors were spared from the plague. It is believed that the chemical nutrients sanitized them as they processed the plants.

Lavender was also used to conceal smells on clothes and in toilets during the middle ages.

As an aromatherapy method, lavender creates a calming effect that can aid in getting you off to sleep. It has properties that calm your digestion helping you to relax as well.

Lavender essential oil sprayed on your pillow at night will help you fall asleep faster, and you will have a more peaceful sleep.

Passionflower: *Passiflora*

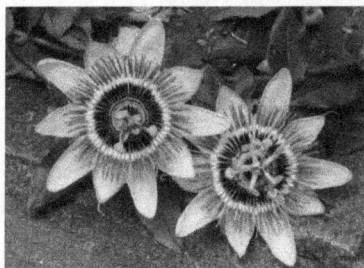

BENEFITS:

Anti-anxiety and stress reliever. Reduces hyperactivity in ADHD patients. Like the above herbs, it slows brain activity allowing you to relax and fall asleep. (GABA; gamma-aminobutyric acid). Mild antioxidant and has been studied for relieving stomach ulcers in rats.

NUTRIENTS:

Vitamins A & C, Potassium, Phosphorus, Magnesium, Iron, Copper.

Passionflower has been grown as a semi-domesticated crop by the Aztecs, Incas & other South American Native people for thousands of years. The plant has been used primarily for its sedative effects. Passionflower can be found on most continents but is native to central America. It is a food source for many varieties of butterfly. Some varieties of passionflower (there are over 500 varieties) have evolved to create small bumps on their leaves that fool butterflies into thinking that eggs have been laid there. That way the butterfly larvae (caterpillar's) won't eat all the vines leaves. Pretty sneaky defense mechanism designed by nature.

Passionflower is primarily used to treat Insomnia and anxiety. However, it is not a great stand-alone herb. It seems to have a more profound effect when combined with other herbs.

Spearmint: *Mentha spicata*

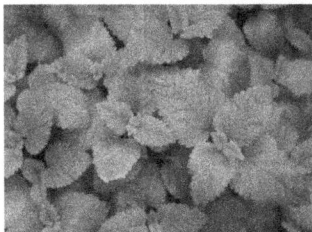

BENEFITS:

Fall asleep with fresh breath and a calmed stomach. Alleviates nausea, is high in antioxidants, and improves memory. May reduce blood pressure, it does reduce stress and anxiety, and can reduce minor aches and pains.

NUTRIENTS:

Vitamins A & C, Potassium, Phosphorus, Magnesium, Manganese, Calcium, Iron.

Most people think of spearmint for its fresh breath feeling. With this blend you will taste a hint of the spearmint, but it is not overpowering. And you'll have fresh breath when you go to sleep. A fun fact: spearmint has been used to remove unwanted hair in the middle east.

Spearmint has antibacterial properties and can clean your mouth. It is high in antioxidants and has been studied, with some success, as a cancer fighting herb. It has also been studied for improving your memory and in one study showed a 15% increase in working memory skills.

Mint is fairly easy to grow in most areas. Having some fresh mint to harvest for fresh breath, calming tea, or added to a recipe is only one of the many benefits. There are over six hundred variations of the mint plant. I have personally grown; chocolate, lemon, apple, pineapple, spearmint, and peppermint. Believe it or not the apple had a subtle apple flavor. This is true of the lemon and pineapple as well. The chocolate tasted like mint. Maybe I did something wrong?

I highly recommend growing your own varieties of mint. It was cool learning about the different flavors of the mint plant. Not only is it easy to grow, but you can also step outside, chew a couple leaves making mint the perfect addition for your night's rest. You may even wake up with fresh breath, your partner, spouse, dog or cat will be happy about that.

CHAMOMILE: Matric aria chamomilla

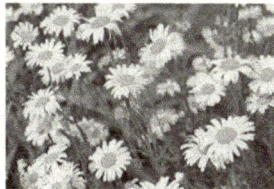

BENEFITS:

Immune system and mood booster, anti-inflammatory, antioxidant, antidepressant, anti-anxiety, it may improve digestion, relaxes the nervous system, lowers blood sugar, and Induces sleep. Calming.

NUTRIENTS:

Vitamin A, Calcium, Potassium, Magnesium, Manganese, Iron, zinc, copper,

Chamomile has been used for centuries like many of the most beneficial plants. It can be traced back to ancient Egypt where it was used in embalming the Pharaohs. In ancient Greece, the noted father of medicine Hippocrates, also mentions chamomile in his writings. Throughout history chamomile has been used as medicine, incense, flavoring, and for fragrance in cosmetics. The word "chamomile" comes from ancient Greece, *Chamomaela*, and means "ground apple". *Pliny the Elder* mentions the similarity of the smell of the chamomile flower to the apple blossom, and this may be why the ancients used the term. The Romans used chamomile to flavor drinks and in incense, as well as a medicinal herb.

The two most popular varieties of chamomile are German and Roman. Roman chamomile is from Western Europe and North Africa, and flowers in late spring or early July. German chamomile is from western Asia, and surprisingly, was used in making beer. German chamomile is more popular and has been studied more extensively, although both versions have good health benefits. Here's a fun fact: Buckingham Palace uses chamomile instead of grass on the grounds.

Chamomile is popular as a calming, sleep promoting herb. A glass or cup o`tea in the evening will help you relax. It should give you a better night's sleep and many people claim they wake up more refreshed the next day after drinking chamomile tea.

TEA HACK:

You may also add a teaspoon of honey for some sweetness. Honey releases serotonin which makes you feel good while falling asleep. Stevia leaves would also add some sweetness as well as other nutrients. (from the Stevia plant, not the synthetic sugar version)

You should not use lemon which may actually wake you up!

Immune Boosting Blend

My favorite immunities building blend creates an environment in your body that promotes healthy cell activity. All the herbs and two berry varieties make this a powerful antioxidant builder that will serve your health well.

Ingredients

- *Elderberry*
- *Ginger*
- *Elder flower*
- *Holy basil (Tulsi)*
- *Blueberry & Blackberry*
- *Lemon peel*

Instructions:

- Blend 1 tsp of each herb into a tea strainer. You can use cheesecloth, or tea bags as well. If filling your own tea bags mix herbs together first, then fill bags with the blend.
- Soak in ½ gallon of water (distilled water is best) for 6 to 12 hours.
- Remove herb packet and serve.

- Makes ½ gallon of tea.

You can use the same herbs for a second soak that will be a little less flavorful. I will sometimes add 2 green or black tea bags during the second soaking to boost flavor and health benefits. *Makes ½ gallon of tea.*Individual tea bags will make 6-8 oz.

Elderberry: *Sambucus*

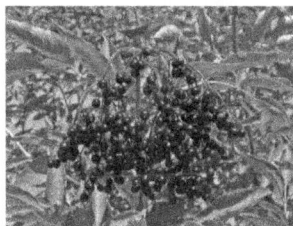

BENEFITS:

High in anthocyanins / antioxidants, fights back hard against diseases. Antiviral, antibacterial, anti-inflammatory, relieves cold and flu symptoms, may also shorten duration of colds. Improves kidney function and relieves stress. Great cold and flu season herb!

NUTRIENTS:

Vitamins A, B6, C, Phosphorus, Magnesium, Calcium, Potassium, Iron.

Throughout history elderberries have been attributed with treating over 70 different maladies from toothaches and fevers to cuts and burns. John Evelyn, a famous 17th century English writer, gardener, and diarist, wrote that if all of the plant's secrets were known, there would not be a disease that couldn't be defeated.

Elderberry has been used to treat influenza, infections, sciatica, headaches, dental pain, heart pain and nerve pain, as well as a laxative and diuretic. One study of 60 people with influenza found that those who took 15 ml of elderberry syrup four times per day showed symptom improvement in two to four days, while the control group took seven to eight days to improve. I can validate this success from personal experience. Elderberry has an amazing way of treating cold and flu symptoms, respiratory issues, and other cold type illnesses.

Another exciting use for elderberries is soaking in honey and then using in cakes and pies. You get a great sweet treat while bringing some awesome health benefits. In my opinion, elderberries, elderberry syrup or a tincture should be in everyone's war chest for good health. They are my go-to source for cold and flu symptom prevention and elimination.

It should be noted that elderberries are poisonous in their raw form. They must be dried or prepared before eating!

Elderflower: *Sambucas*

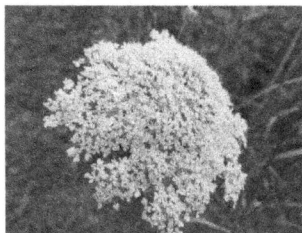

BENEFITS:

Relieves flu symptoms, reduces Influenza symptoms, is high in antioxidants. It is an antiviral, antibacterial, anti-inflammatory, antiseptic. Like elderberries this herb will help alleviate cold and flu symptoms.

NUTRIENTS:

Vitamins A, B6, C, Phosphorus, Magnesium, Calcium, Potassium, Iron

Amazingly, in studies in 2006, an extract from the elderberry plant (berries, leaves and stems) was proven to be effective against the H5N1 strain of avian flu. (bird flu, swine flu) This fascinating plant has been helping humans heal for millennia. Archeologists have uncovered bodies from prior to the pre-Egyptian era (10,000 - 40,000 years ago) with elderberry/elderflower tincture next to the bodies. Apparently, the benefits of elderberry have been known since the beginning of time.

Renowned British herbalist Maude Grieve wrote in the 1930's about the elderflower and its use as "one of the best preventatives known against the advance of influenza and the ill-effects of a chill".

You cannot find a better antiviral natural plant. Utilizing the whole elderberry plant in this blend, is going to send your immune system soaring to the moon.

Ginger:

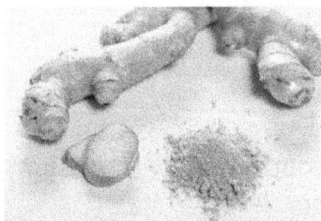

BENEFITS:
Antiviral, anti-bacterial, anti-inflammatory, anti-nausea. Ginger improves circulation, lowers blood sugar, and is loaded with antioxidants. Ginger has been used in Chinese medicine for thousands of years as an immunity booster.

NUTRIENTS:

Vitamin B6, & C, Potassium, Magnesium. Manganese,

Ginger gets its name from the Sanskrit word "srngaveram" which means "horn body". This refers to the roots, or rhizomes, and they do look kind of horny. Ginger has its roots in Asia; however, it can be found around the world today.

Thought of as a spice primarily, ginger has been used medicinally for thousands of years. It can be found in the writings of most ancient mid-eastern and Asian cultures. It has been used in Ayurvedic medicine as an anti-inflammatory agent and to treat indigestion, nausea, stomachache toothache, insomnia, flatulent intestinal colic, respiratory and urinary tract infections, rheumatism, diabetes, infertility, nervous diseases, morning sickness, cold and flu, as well as to strengthen the memory.

Ginger, orange juice, turmeric and a dash of honey make an excellent cold and flu immune booster. Fill a shot glass with the ingredients and take itb2 or 3 times a day. You will be amazed at the healing benefits.

Tulsi (Holy Basil):

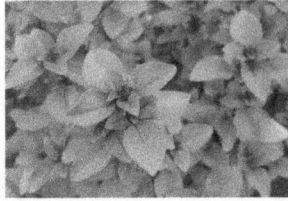

BENEFITS:

Balances the body while promoting optimal health. Antimicrobial, antibacterial, antiviral, antifungal and more, antidiarrheal, Antioxidant, Anti-inflammatory, Liver, brain and heart protectant, Antidiabetic, Antipyretic, Antitussive, (treats cough), Anti-arthritic, Anti-coagulant, Apoptogenic, stress reducer and more. Just an amazing life-giving herb.

NUTRIENTS:

Vitamins A, C, & K. Iron, Calcium, Zinc. Manganese.
Dried Tulsi has 43% RDA of vitamin K, whereas fresh basil has approximately 5%.

Holy basil is one of the few herbs that I use almost every day. The variety of nutrients in the plant brings health to every area of your body. It is my favorite balancing herb for this reason. It is an apoptogenic herb that reduces stress and anxiety while building your immune system. Promotes a healthy gut by strengthening the stomach lining. It balances blood sugar, reduces bad cholesterol, improves memory, is food for the eyes and improves cognitive abilities. Wow, what an amazing herb.

Tulsi can be grown easily indoors near a window or grow light. In warmer climates zone 9b and above holy basil can be grown outdoors with little effort. I grow copious amounts of basil in an aquaponics set up on my patio. I harvest several times a year, filling a quart sized mason jar after drying and grinding after each harvest. This is one herb I feel needs to be always on hand.

As a sacred herb the Hindu religion places holy basil on a pedestal, and knowing how this herb totally balances the body, I feel it is sacred myself. Try adding a teaspoon to your tea at least once a day for two weeks. I believe you will feel healthier, more alert, and calm. What an amazing herb.

Blueberries & Blackberries:

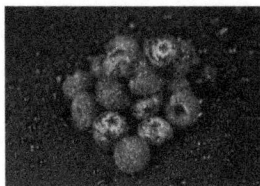

BENEFITS:
Antioxidant, anti-inflammatory, anticancer, improves cardiovascular system, can prevent type 2 diabetes, improves brain functions, may reduce/prevent Alzheimer's disease,

NUTRIENTS:

Vitamins A, C, B6, Potassium, Magnesium, Iron,

Not an herb, I know. However, these berries should be in our diets every day when possible. Adding them to a tea is another way for the body to absorb the amazing antioxidant, anticancer benefits. As well as a plentiful supply of vitamins and minerals

One study showed that blueberries, blackberries, and raspberries have the highest antioxidant activity of commonly consumed fruits, with pomegranates having the most. What do antioxidants do? They fight free radicals (zombie cells) which can increase cancers in your body. More antioxidants, less cancer. Berries are loaded with cancer fighting nutrients. Berries also contain high amounts of *anthocyanins* that are believed to have preventative and therapeutic properties, such as the ability to lower the risk of cardiovascular disease and stroke.

Here IS A really cool Fruit Hack:

Take your Blueberries and freeze them at least twenty-four hours before eating. The frozen berries become super sweet. I've looked everywhere for the reason and have come up empty. Trust me I don't know the science behind it, but frozen blueberries are sweeter than fresh.

Lemon or lemon peel: *Citrus Limon*

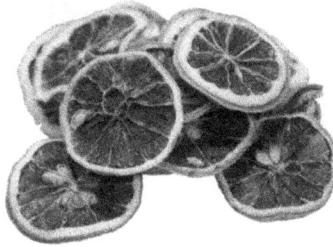

BENEFITS:

antiviral, antibacterial, anti-inflammatory, antifungal, antimicrobial,

NUTRIENTS:

Vitamin A, C, E, Potassium, Phosphorus, Zinc, Magnesium, Iron, Calcium.

Lemon peel will give your system a little energy boost, while providing vitamin C and other needed minerals. Lemons contain the terpene, limonene which assists in providing a healthy environment in your body, as well as giving the lemon it's fresh scent.

Lemon use has been documented since the first century, however its use is believed to be much older. Originating in India, lemons were brought to North America by Christopher Columbus in 1493.

Around 20 million tons of lemons are harvested annually with most of them coming from India, Mexico, and China. The United States produces around a million tons of lemons annually. In case you were wondering, one lemon tree can produce around 600 pounds of lemons a year.

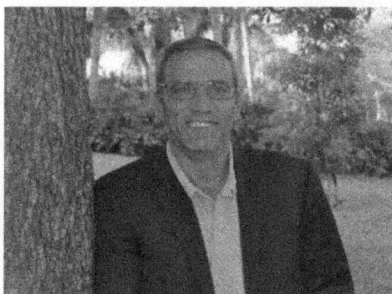

Balanced By Nature

What does it mean to be balanced by nature? The simple answer is eat and medicate naturally, maintain positive momentum, be grateful, and embrace nature. Those four lifegiving attitudes will guarantee you good health and happiness. When you are healthy and happy your level of abundance can only increase.

I have spent over ten years growing and medicating with fruits, vegetables, and herbs including cannabis. I learned what nutrients the plants needed and how the plant's environment affected how the plant grew. I also used my growing knowledge to grow fruit, vegetables, and herbs on my own 16'x16' urban patio garden. Learning about plant nutrient needs piqued my interest in nutrient needs for our bodies and minds. After extensive self-study I realized the plants generally provide the perfect assortment of natural nutrients to balance our bodies. While synthetic medicines and processed foods alter our bodies requiring you to take additional synthetic products to balance the unnatural effects.

I have researched over several years, how nature, plants, and positivity can heal our bodies. I discovered that we have three life centers in our body, and most fruits, vegetables, and herbs benefit all three centers.

Using this knowledge, I was able to create a plan to eliminate synthetic drugs and begin to feel more balanced in life. With a mostly natural-food diet you can stay away from most sickness. When you do get sick, medicating with nature will heal you without creating deadly side effects. I have not had a synthetic pharmaceutical drug since 2016. Herbal tea has been a major influence in my good health. I hope it will be for you as well.

Stephen T Radentz

Stephen is available to share his journey and insights with your organization.

For more information, contact him at:
Steve@balancedbynature.net,

www.ingramcontent.com/pod-product-compliance
Lightning Source LLC
Chambersburg PA
CBHW020521030426

42337CB00011B/506